Ignite Your Inner Healer

Transformational Tools to Heal Your Body, Mind and Soul

Ana Marinho

This book is being given to

_____

Because I care about you and
your greater health

_____

Praise for
Ignite Your Inner Healer

Ignite Your Inner Healer is a well-written and thought-provoking introduction to alternative healing and wellness. The author's method of reading through and then slowly working with each chapter is a sound one, and I liked having access to a workbook designed for the text. Her ideas for pain management are particularly interesting and have proven to be useful since I've begun using them. Anyone who's wondered why the so-called 'magic cures' promoted by the pharmaceutical industry don't seem to be working all that well should take a look at this book and discover how they might play a larger role in their personal healing journey. *Ignite Your Inner Healer*: Transformational Tools to Heal Your Body, Mind and Soul is most highly recommended.

- Reviewed By Jack Magnus for Readers' Favorite (five stars)

I feel incredibly empowered and hopeful after reading Ana's book. She brings about an incredibly refreshing angle to health in a way that is revolutionary. Ana brings science, research, psychology and movement to the table, and not only shows us how they intertwine themselves, but how we can practically use them in unique ways to substantially improve our holistic health.

- Chad Kuntz | physical therapist
www.pr1memovement.com

Ignite Your Inner Healer is engaging, informative and easy to read. I recommend it to those looking to achieve personal growth and optimize on wellness. I truly enjoyed this book and am able to put these valuable learning tools into practice in my daily life!

- Ashley Friend | physical therapist

Ignite Your Inner Healer is a revolutionary practical guide that will help you change thought processes that are holding you back from living your best life. Ana utilizes scientific research as well as her own clinical experiences to help teach the reader how to heal themselves from the mental blocks that are most likely adding to their pain, whether that pain is on the body level, mind level or emotional/spiritual.

You will walk away from this book feeling empowered, wiser, healthier, and more optimistic. Your health, your healing and your limitless possibilities are all within reach and *Ignite Your Inner Healer* will show you how.

One of my favorite aspects within this book is the practical tools that I was able to apply immediately to my daily life with ease. It has been a true delight to observe the positive changes the tools I gained by reading this book have had on my life, my family and my patients.

This is a must-read book for all healthcare professionals, all pain-sufferers and anyone hoping to break through the walls of emotional suffering to lead an inspired and purposeful life.

- Marissa J. Moshonisiotis | acupuncturist
www.mdholistichealth.com

Ana takes the complexities of neuroscience and the mind-body connection and breaks them down into incredibly simple and easy-to-do steps that will create major shifts when utilized. As a student of these principles and concepts for many years in my career, and someone who has dealt with chronic illness, I can attest both personally and professionally to the quality content within this book!

- Holly Joy McCabe | Fitness, wellness and mindset coaching, retreats and plant-based health
www.spiritualfitchick.com

This is a great, insightful dive into learning more about ourselves as humans, but more importantly, how we can look inwards and utilize our own healing abilities to live our best lives. I highly recommend this book for anyone who is serious about their own health and wellness!

- Dave Kittle | physical therapist
www.ConciergePainRelief.com
www.CashBasedPhysicalTherapy.org

This book provides helpful information about the mind/body connection and includes practical tools for quieting your mind and connecting to your body in a deeper way. These tools can help you address the health issues you are experiencing and move forward with greater awareness to create healthier habits within all aspects of your life.

- Kerri McManus | conscious creativity coach
www.kerrimcmanus.com

Ignite your Inner Healer offers breakthrough insights for those wanting to, and ready to, take responsibility for their own health and well-being. Ana Marinho, through her coaching and therapeutic background as a health-care provider, brings together science and simplicity, making sense of a self-healing path that is often presented in complicated and heavy-to-read books.

If you are serious about the health of your mind and body, this book you hold in your hands may prove the perfect stepping stone. Inspiring, engaging and so very useful in a world where so many seekers do not know where to begin — as a fellow health practitioner, I found this book incredibly refreshing, informative and honest.
- **Diya Welland**| evolutionary coach
and neurological bodyworker

Whether you are just beginning your healing journey or are many years in, *Ignite Your Inner Healer* offers valuable lessons to return to again and again. Ana's compassion and genuine desire to guide you on your journey comes through in every page of this book.
- **Tamara Sullivan** | Reiki master, bioenergetics, yoga, meditation and sound therapy
Facebook page: Centered Spirit

I loved that this book is short and easy to read, yet contains all of the tools required to experience profound healing physically, mentally and emotionally. I have worked with Ana for several weeks, and she helped me uncover the causes of my chronic back pain. We used the tools in this book, and gradually my pain diminished. Today, I am pain-free. I now understand that the power to "ignite my inner healer" was with me all along and I will gratefully embrace and nurture this awareness for the rest of my life!

- Sheila Crane | AFAA certified fitness instructor and RYT 500 registered yoga teacher
Facebook page: <u>One Love Yoga</u>

A fantastic read for those that are curious. Simple and easy to read with practical exercises that on the surface seem simple. However, when applied to your daily routine provide amazing results. I applaud anyone who uses their curiosity to discover their truth. Be curious! Live with intention and amazing things will happen. This is the perfect tool to unlock the gateway to your truth and start your journey in the care of Ana.

- Michelle Campbell |transition coach
Facebook page: <u>Life Began</u>

Acknowledgments

This book is dedicated to:

- My patients and clients

All of you have inspired me to ask unconventional questions and ignited my curiosity to research beyond the ordinary. Every session that I offer is an opportunity to learn more about the interconnectedness of the body, mind and soul.

- My family, friends, mentors and coaches

You allow me to be myself and explore my gifts, even when they are outside of the norm. I am also grateful for all the challenging questions that have guided me to discover who I am.

- My husband, Chris

Thank you for believing in me unconditionally, for being my friend, my confidant, my support and my partner.

- You, the reader

I also thank you. Without you, writing this book would be a waste. I am so glad that you are ready to take ownership of your health.

CONTENTS

FOREWORD

In 1987, I was a vibrant young woman fresh out of college and fully engaged in all that life had to offer me. In 1988, I was taking care of my beloved father as he endured chemotherapy and radiation and rapidly declined from lung cancer.

During this time, I started having severe digestive issues. I was diagnosed with Crohn's disease and was told it was incurable. Confused as to why this suddenly happened to me while all my friends had no health issues, I asked my physician what caused it. Was it the stress of my father's fate? He told me that the medical community did not know what the cause was, but they definitely knew it was not from stress.

Even at the tender age of 24, I could not believe my state of mind was not a factor in my chronic condition. After struggling for a year taking toxic drugs I had severe reactions to, I said, "Enough!" I had a talk with God and emphatically said if it is my destiny to be sick, then I accept it, but I am going to enjoy my life anyway and stop taking these drugs. Period.

When I woke up in the morning, my digestion was completely normal and my 'incurable' disease was 100 percent gone. I could not believe it! By making peace in my mind, I had healed myself.

The gift of that spontaneous healing eventually propelled me to become a yoga therapist and an Ayurveda wellness practitioner. These ancient sciences acknowledge that disease starts in the mind from the inability to digest life experiences.

My work is dedicated to helping my clients understand this, and so is Ana's. Though she is an extremely gifted physical therapist, Ana's magic lies in her ability to discern intuitively which mental/emotional blockages are at the root of her clients' issues. She gently guides them to understand the origin of their disease so they are empowered to regain balance on all levels.

From my own personal sessions with her, I can attest that Ana's skills are truly unparalleled — she is a master healer. And the clients I have referred to her have experienced amazing clarity and transformation very quickly.

Ignite Your Inner Healer is a must-read for anyone who wants to get off the medical merry-go-round of merely treating symptoms and confidently take control of their health.

The book offers a simple, powerful, step-by-step process to tune in easily to the wisdom of the body and to harness our thoughts so they may work for us and not against us. Rewiring the brain is key to our personal power and success and Ana teaches us that it is actually quite accessible.

Ignite Your Inner Healer

Spontaneous healings are readily available to all of us and Ignite Your Inner Healer offers the tools to tap into that innate ability that we are all born with.

- Lisa Moore | certified yoga therapist,
Ayurveda wellness practitioner,
200/300/500 Hour Ayur-therapeutic
yoga teacher training
www.HarmonyYogaNC.com

Charlotte, NC

FREE WORKBOOK

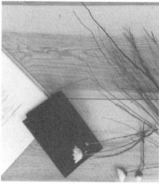

Download your FREE workbook now

There are many tools and many different ways that we can amplify the power of self-healing. The tools presented in this book are only a few that you can play with. I hope you enjoy this journey of self-discovery as much as my clients do.

To amplify the power of your process, download your FREE *Ignite Your Inner Healer* workbook at (www.behealthywithana.com/workbook)

This step-by-step guide helps you practice the techniques outlined inside the book, allowing you to achieve mastery and track your progress every step of the way. It is the perfect reference journal to have at your fingertips.

1

HOW TO USE THIS BOOK

Healing is like peeling an onion, or the slow blossoming of an exquisite flower. I believe that healing happens in layers or stages. Each layer is needed to make it to the next layer. Each piece that we learn about ourselves is instrumental for the next step of the journey.

This book is a step-by-step process.

Each chapter will take you deeper; each chapter will allow you to *Ignite Your Inner Healer* more and more.

I suggest you read through the book once.

Then read it again slowly, taking your time to answer each question and apply each chapter to your life. This book contains transformational tools and many powerful questions within each chapter.

You will be surprised how much you will learn about yourself and your health.

I also recommend you start a journal where you can record your answers and insights. You can download the *Ignite Your Inner Healer* workbook at www.behealthywithana.com/workbook; in it you can write your answers as you read the book.

Nature has no resistance.

You just add a seed in the soil, a little bit of water, some sun and it will sprout. Nature has so much to teach.

This book is like a seed.

You can choose to place your seed in the sun or the shade, and how much water you will give it, etc.

You can choose to treat this book as just another book, or you can choose to explore each exercise and each chapter with an open heart and truly grow.

Even better, share this journey with a friend to create accountability or create a group. Then you can have fun and share your answers with each other.

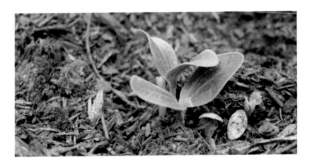

How much will you grow?

How much will you learn about yourself?
How deep will you go?
It is totally up to you!

I hope you choose to learn more about yourself and let this book transform your health.

Even if you have heard all the information contained within this book before, until you are actually applying it in your life, then you do not really *know* it yet.

Be open to **seeing with different lenses**.
Be open to **trying something new**.
Be open to **taking actions**.
Be open to **finding yourself**.

I am delighted to share this journey with you.
I am overjoyed that you will share your journey with me.
Enjoy the ride.

Let this seed sprout in your heart!

Common Benefits

These tools may look simple. If, however, you practice the exercises offered, they will transform your life. In my practice, I have seen these powerful tools change people's health.

As you start to read this book and practice the exercises in each chapter, benefits may include:

- experiencing less daily stress;
- decreasing your aches and pains;
- increasing your healing speed;
- boosting your self-confidence;
- achieving more mental clarity;
- establishing a deeper bodily connection;
- reducing your negative thoughts.

**You might not believe it yet, but it is
absolutely possible and
you absolutely deserve it.**

Everyone has a doctor
in him or her.
We just have to help it in its work.
The natural healing force within
each one of us is the greatest force
in getting well.

Hippocrates

A patient woke up one day in a hospital bed after an accident. The doctors told him that he would **never walk again**. He refused to believe that would be his new reality.

Every day, as he lay in the hospital bed, he started to visualize his toes moving; however, nothing happened. He did not give up. He knew that the **body can heal when given the right tools**.

One day his toes actually moved. It was a long journey and he used all the tools that he could.

Now, when **he walks into the office** using a cane, he says:

> **"If I can do that,
> everyone can do that too."**

2

IS IT POSSIBLE TO HEAL YOURSELF?

The body is created to self-heal.

If we cut ourselves, the cut will stop bleeding, close, and repair itself even if you do not use anything on it, right?

If a cell dies, another cell is created. In fact, cells are always created and destroyed in the human body. About 300 million cells die every minute in our bodies! (UCSB, 2013)

The body knows exactly what to do.

The ability to heal is intrinsic to all multicellular organisms. This is an incredible ability that the plant and animal kingdoms attained through evolution (Cremaldi & Bhushan, 2018).

Humans are no different. The concept of the body as a self-healing organism is not new. In fact, it has been around as long as people have been treating illnesses. Ancient healers from around the world noted that given enough time and support, the body will often correct itself (Milner, 2018).

You may ask: Why am I not healing?

Well, something caused your body to forget those skills. However, you are not alone.

Today, Americans are taking more medications than ever before. Nearly 60 to 70 percent take at least one prescribed drug. Recent analysis estimates 128,000 Americans die each year as a result of taking medications as prescribed (Milner, 2018) (Schroeder, 2016).

In 2016, U.S. Centers for Medicare & Medicaid Services reported that the U.S. health care spending increased 4.3 percent to reach $10,348 per person (U.S. Centers for Medicare & Medicaid Services, 2016).

The good news is you do not have to be part of that statistic. It is possible to have good health. It is possible to *ignite your inner healer* and to heal whatever you are dealing with right now, whether it is physical, emotional, and/or spiritual.

I see that happen in my office every day. Someone walks in with excruciating pain, limping around, feeling depressed and hopeless and in a few sessions, the body heals and the person is pain-free and happy again.

I experienced that happening in my own body too.

I was in my mid 20s when I was diagnosed with cervical dysplasia (a stage before cancer). Dysplasia is the presence of abnormal cells within a tissue; it is when the body starts to reproduce damaged cells, instead of healthy cells.

I was shocked. I was frustrated. I was terrified. I considered myself healthy. Nevertheless, the reality was I had no idea what 'healthy' really was.

I could not stop saying to myself, "My grandma died from cancer. I am way too young to die. I am way too young to deal with pre-cancer."

The doctor wanted to do an invasive procedure to freeze cells in my uterus. This would kill the precancerous cells (and the healthy cells too). The doctor hoped that, following the procedure, the precancerous cells would not return.

I asked the doctor, "Why is this happening? What can I do to prevent the precancerous cells from returning?" She did not have an answer.

I refused the traditional treatment and started a deep quest.

I wanted to know why my body was creating so many unhealthy cells to begin with.

I started to research about self-healing and the mind-body connection.

I went to a holistic nutritionist, to an acupuncturist, to an energy healer, a health coach and every other health professional that gave me a drop of hope. Finally, I realized I was the one creating the unhealthy cells, and I was the only person that had the power to stop it from happening again.

The reality is our bodies change every day. Every day new cells are born and old cells die. Every day, we either hold stress in our bodies or we allow our bodies to relax.

Every action, every food, every thought, every emotion is either helping us to be healthier or causing us to be sicker.

A balanced body creates healthy and happy cells while clearing away the weaker and sicker cells. This is normal physiology. It is part of the body's healing mechanism.

When the body is not in balance, it starts to do the opposite. It kills the healthy cells and reproduces the weak or sick cells. Stress, worries, fear, anger, negative feelings and/or thoughts, poor nutrition, lack of exercise, lack of sleep, etc. will cause the body to get out of balance.

On the other hand, eating a healthy diet, exercising, having a good night's sleep, being in nature, practicing meditation, gratitude and self-awareness, and many other things will help your body to feel better.

But you probably heard that before.

Let me share with you some of the research that I found during my quest and some of the practical techniques that I used to restore my own health — with no doctors and with no drugs.

HOW DOES THE BODY HEAL ITSELF?

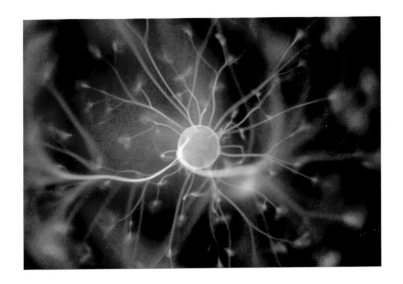

3

YOU CAN REWIRE YOUR BRAIN

Habits play an important role in our health.

Understanding the science behind habit development, and learning how we can break bad habits and create new ones can help us to make healthier choices.

The research on neuroplasticity (the brain's ability to reorganize itself by forming new neural connections throughout life) shows that we are very capable of creating new pathways through practice and repetition no matter how old we are.

Neuron patterns (habits, belief systems, thoughts) are like rivers.

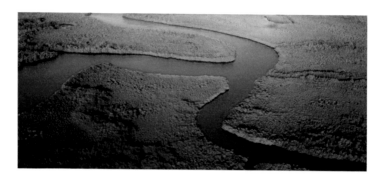

The water always travels the same course unless it is forced in a new direction, perhaps by a fallen tree, rock or dam. After being redirected, the water forges new courses. This pattern is very much how thoughts travel in our brain.

When we learn a new habit, we continue the same pattern until something or someone challenges us to move in a new direction. Some habits are old (formed when we were a child), and others are new (developed recently as a result of some stimulus, such as adopting the latest diet after watching the news).

Some habits promote self-healing and others inhibit your body from healing. Over time, if we reinforce the poor habits, we can forge deep and familiar pathways in our brains, making it difficult to navigate in a different direction.

Poor habits can be physical (unhealthy diet, lack of sleep, lack of exercise and poor posture are some examples) or emotional (negative self-talk, overreacting, self-doubt, feeling guilty, perfectionism and so on).

We can change our poor habits.

The good news is that no matter how long ago they were established, we can change each of the poor habits that impact our well-being.

Are you ready to create new pathways?

It is an old, commonly held belief that once we reach adulthood our brains are 'hard-wired' and incapable of dramatic change. However, research in recent years has led neuroscientists to believe that our brains are in fact much more malleable, flexible and able to shift physically and psychologically than we first thought (Swart, 2018).

The research on neuroplasticity shows that with practice, we can train our brains to choose new pathways (Swart, 2018).

Eventually, the road less traveled begins to become the road most traveled, ultimately leading us toward more positive outcomes.

How cool is that?

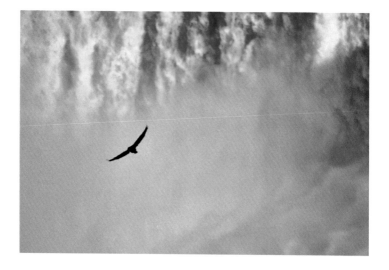

4

IS YOUR CUP HALF FULL OR HALF EMPTY?

You have probably heard that expression before. You may even know that this question relates to how people see the world around them.

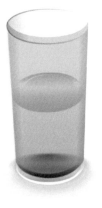

Some people see the cup as half full. They have optimistic thinking characterized by the belief that the future is full of hope and opportunities to be successful. They focus on sentences like

"What if...?"
"I can..."
"I know I am capable of..."

Optimistic thinkers believe that negative events are caused by external factors, and that they are isolated exceptions to the rule. When something bad happens, people who think optimistically believe that it is not something that will reoccur (unstable), they are not responsible for the bad event (external event), and the event has a limited effect (specific) (Williams, 2018).

> For example, M.B. is a marathon runner, she believes that she did not finish the race (bad outcome) because it was too hot, which is an external factor. She believes that she will receive a gold medal at the next marathon, which indicates that M.B believes that her failure is an unstable event that will not likely reoccur. She also believes that her failure is a specific, isolated event ("I will not fail again").

Optimistic thinking is beneficial because it improves your self-esteem, your ability to handle stress, your mood, your ability to recuperate from sickness as well as your overall mental and physical health (Williams, 2018). Optimistic thinkers' brains are wired to be more positive, they are healthier and happier, and they see possibilities everywhere.

The brains of pessimistic thinkers are wired to see the cup as half empty when they are faced with a challenging situation. Pessimistic thinking is characterized by the belief that bad things are a common occurrence and that there is little hope for the future (Williams, 2018). Pessimistic thinkers focus on negative thoughts and limit possibilities and opportunities.

Sometimes pessimistic people live their lives holding back on pursuing their dreams. Sometimes they even lack the ability to dream. They usually focus on sentences like

"I can't..."
"I'm not capable of..."
"It's impossible..."
"If only this happens, then I can..."
"I can't feel better. I will feel this pain forever."
"If only I had more energy, then I would heal."
"No matter how much I try, nobody can help me."

> If M.B. were a pessimist, she would have likely attributed her failure to her poor running abilities (internal), and believed that her abilities would prevent her from continuing to do well in future marathons (stable), and that she will continue to be unsuccessful in other endeavors as well (global).

What have you been focusing on lately?

No matter what your answer is, you can always train your brain to be more efficient.

If you are feeling any pain or dealing with any physical or emotional challenge, chances are that you have been using your pessimistic neuron pathways.

Ana Marinho

Positive Thinking vs. Optimism vs. Pessimism

How do optimism and positive thinking differ? Is optimism not a kind of positive thinking?

The way we separate the two is by definition — positive thinking is a broad range of hypotheses, theories and practices, while optimism can be defined as hopefulness and confidence about the future or the success of something. Even if someone thinks negatively, it is possible for them to still be optimistic (CBHS, 2017).

A typical example would be someone that is overweight and suffering from diabetes.

The optimistic thinker would acknowledge the extra weight and diabetes as issues, but have hope or confidence that circumstances can change for the better. They are more likely to face those problems and commit to diet and exercise leading to better physical and mental health.

A positive thinker, on the other hand, may say, "Everything is fine, my health is fine, everything will resolve itself if I am positive." They may or may not take actions and they may not even believe what they are saying to themselves.

The challenge with positive thinking is that a lot of people try very hard to see the good in everything, but inside they are fighting with themselves because their brains are not wired that way yet. Until you feel it, hear it, taste it, smell it and see it, positive thinking may not work for you. The body needs a whole-body experience using all our five senses to believe and transform the brain. The body sometimes needs more than just thinking positively; it needs action.

On the other hand, the pessimist might have a completely opposite experience — perhaps recognizing the threat but not acting on it — because often they do not believe that it is possible to have a positive outcome even if they try.

Optimism and pessimism are both necessary for our survival and wellness.

Nonetheless, the literature suggests that, in regard to one's general attitude, being in the middle of the optimism-pessimism continuum is not necessarily the best (Hecht, 2013).

A moderate dose of optimism can be advantageous.

Studies that investigated the correlation between optimism and health suggest that optimists generally have better physical health, fewer cardiovascular diseases and improved immunological functioning (Hecht, 2013).

Optimistic Mindset	Pessimistic Mindset
Opportunity is everywhere and I can train myself to see it.	I do not see opportunity; therefore, it does not exist.
If there is one person in the world who has done it, then so can I.	I create a list of reasons why I cannot achieve what I want.
Most people have good intentions.	People are terrible and they do not treat me well.
I find solutions.	I find problems.
Some things come easy, others require a bit more effort.	Things should be easy and I resent that they are not.
Failures and setbacks mean I have moved forward and grown.	Failures and setbacks mean that my self-doubt must be true.

Many times, I hear from patients with chronic pain

"I will never feel better."
"If only I were pain-free, then I'd be happy."

What if you *could* be happy even before you are pain-free?
What if feeling happier helps to heal your pain?

Being optimistic opens a new door to solutions beyond your imagination.

Optimism is like a child that climbs a tree and wonders about the view.
She is curious.
She is courageous.
She is confident.
She believes in herself.

You can rewire your brain and be optimistic about your health (and also your life).

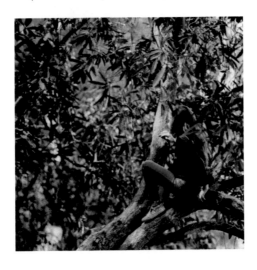

Ana Marinho

HOW CAN I REWIRE MY BRAIN?

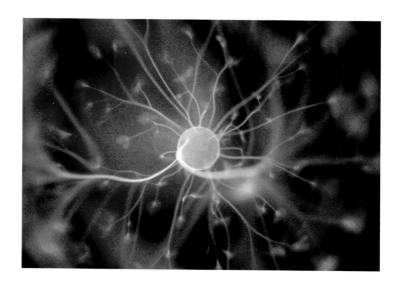

Exercise: Seeing with Different Lenses

Every day, for one week, identify any thoughts that draw energy away from what you truly desire.

1. Notice the negative thoughts.

Notice all the thoughts and beliefs that are holding you back; any pessimistic thoughts like

> "I can't..."
> "This will not work..."
> "If only I could..."
> "It's impossible..."

2. Calm the thought.

Focus on your breath, and take five deep breaths.

Visualize yourself seated in your favorite place. Perhaps you can imagine yourself overlooking a lake or your favorite beach.

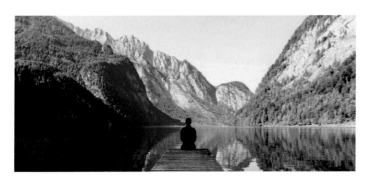

3. Release the judgment.

Once you feel relaxed and safe, let the negative thoughts come to the surface without judging yourself.

Remember that those thoughts were habits created to protect you. Somehow, your body believed that those negative thoughts were the most efficient and safe neuropathway. Now it is time to be grateful for those habits that allowed you to survive until today and let them know that you are ready to create new pathways.

You can say to those thoughts something like

"Yes, I see you. I hear you. I see that you're just trying to keep me safe. Thank you. But I will take it from here. I am ready to create new habits and new thought patterns. I've got this."

4. Be curious.

Now that you have embraced and released the negative thoughts, you can create new ones. You can ask questions like these (use all five of your senses, or as many senses as possible):

> What if I can...?
> What if it does work?
> What if I could improve my health?
> What if I can be pain-free?
> What if I can feel happier and have more energy?
> What if I can create more time for myself?

What if I find a way to do it all?
What if I could live a normal life?
What if I can say "No" to the things that harm my soul?
What if I can feel stronger?
What if I can walk better?
What if I can sleep better?
What if...

You can choose to see the world full of possibilities instead of fears.

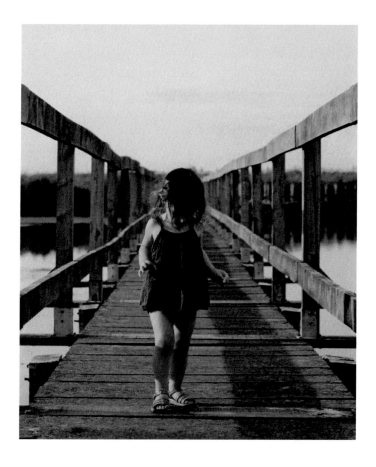

5. Ask with a sense of possibility.

Ask with curiosity, just like a little child. Ask with true wonder.

Be open to seeing with different lenses.
Be open to trying something new.
Be open to taking actions.
Be open to finding yourself.

Notice how you feel.

Does that not feel more powerful?

Well done! You have just created a big opening for creative inspiration, new ideas/insights, new possibilities and self-healing to come in.

Watch for it.
Listen for it.
Ignite it.
Thank it.
Act on it.

> Wonder is the beginning of wisdom.
>
> Socrates

5

BODY WISDOM

Once we start to change our mindset and start to believe that **yes, it is possible**, we can find out **HOW** it is possible!

Our body knows exactly what we need and when we need it.

Our body has all the answers.

The biggest challenge is that we are influenced by our friends, family, the media, etc. — everyone thinks they know what you should eat, do, be. We grow up in a society that ignores our body wisdom.

What is body wisdom?

Body wisdom is that sense of knowing; that message that we receive from our body informing us of what we need. Some people describe this as intuition. With experience, however, we come to know that body wisdom adds an extra dimension to intuition.

For example, when our bodies need extra energy, we feel hungry. When we need to eliminate toxins, we start to sweat, or we feel the need to go to the bathroom.

Some of these messages are crucial for survival; others can safely be ignored or postponed.

For example, if you go on a hike, after a while, your body starts to feel tired and starts to give you signs that you are close to your limit. Those messages are usually like a whisper, a soft voice in your ear. If you decide to push through because you really want to see that beautiful view of the sunset from the top of the mountain, your body may start to 'scream' at you. That scream can be a sensation, such as a pain, spasm or cramp of a muscle, swelling, shortness of breath, or exhaustion. Those sensations can be mild or severe depending on how much you ignore the signals from your body.

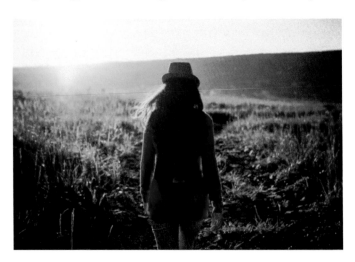

Our body is an astonishing machine and has evolved to tolerate and adapt to a lot of different situations. That is why athletes continue to break world records.

Body wisdom is how our body communicates. It is the way that our body keeps us healthy and safe. It is the way athletes know how far to push themselves.

What would happen if we turn off that wisdom?

Think about when you were a child and your body asked you to move, run, or jump, but you were taught to ignore that feeling and sit still (for hours).

Now, as an adult, you have learned to ignore that signal that the brain was sending, and you end up sitting for hours every day. You learned to ignore that signal that the brain was sending. Messages like "It is time to move" or "I am feeling stiff" and the knowledge that "this will hurt" are dismissed every day.

And we wonder why so many people have back pain.

We learn to tolerate the discomfort. We learn that pain is part of life. The more we tolerate discomfort or pain, the more our brains start to change their physiology and adapt to this new reality. Neuroplasticity works for bad habits too, right?

Well, when we learn to ignore the messages from our bodies, we can fall into a rabbit hole. With time, our body wisdom becomes a whisper far away, and it is often very hard even to acknowledge (or feel) that it still exists.

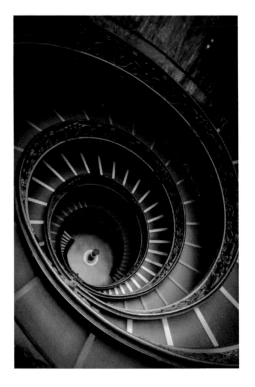

The more distant we are from our body's perceptions, the more disconnected we become from that wisdom.

As we lose that wisdom, it is easier to do what someone else says we should do. Ultimately, we lose the connection with what works for us.

How many times have you followed advice, a diet, an exercise routine, etc. to find out that it did not work for you at all?

Did you check in with your body wisdom before saying "Yes" to that?

Asking for help

It is alright to ask for help when the body cannot provide answers.

A heart attack does not develop in a day or even a month. Imagine how many times someone ignored their body wisdom before the body crashed.

Sometimes, that body wisdom is so distant. You have been trying to heal on your own for so long without success that you will need extra support to heal your body.

You may need to search for help.

You can use your body wisdom to guide you to a professional that can help you. That professional could be a doctor, a physical therapist, an acupuncturist, life coach, healer, etc.

Your body can guide you to find the *best* doctor, physical therapist, acupuncturist, life coach or healer for *you*.

Sometimes, Western medicine, medication and surgeries are necessary. If you need that kind of extra help, that is not wrong.

Try as hard as you can to find a solution for your problem, not just a 'Band-Aid'. You deserve a solution that will allow your body to improve its healing abilities and not just mask the pain temporarily.

You can ask your doctor questions such as these:
Why am I having this problem?
Why is it happening on my right side and not on my left?
How can we prevent this from happening again in the future?

Ask questions, clarify, and ask again.

You deserve to find a professional that listens to you; someone that is knowledgeable, warm and engaged in your care.

Once you have a proper diagnosis (consequence) and understand why that happened (cause), then you can create a proper plan.

Be careful with any plan that is created without knowing what caused the problem. Remember pains, cramps, spasms, swelling, etc. are the consequence. Until we correct the cause, the body will continue to whisper at you. One day it may start to scream again.

That is why so many people have surgery and do not feel the relief they expect. Many studies suggest that common surgeries sometimes do very little for some patients (Belluck, 2013).

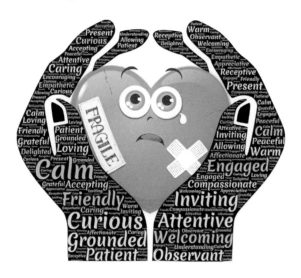

Make sure that you find a health care provider that will find the cause of the problem, and will also provide extra tools to boost your healing abilities, while also honoring your inner wisdom.

Most people are not even aware that it is possible to find out what is better for them before making a decision.

Most people have never heard that the body talks; that it gives us messages about our well-being. If you are one of these people, the next question is...

Ana Marinho

HOW CAN I TAP INTO MY BODY'S WISDOM?

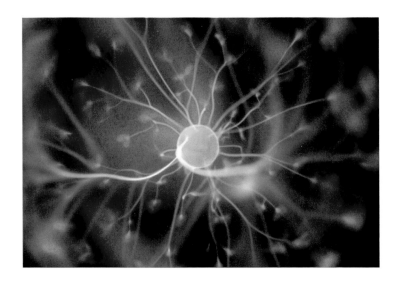

Exercise: Connecting with Your Body

Every day, for one week, sit comfortably in a quiet place.
Notice how you are feeling.
Notice how your body feels.

1. Observe yourself and your body.

Bring attention to the areas of your health that you would like to improve. Notice how you feel about those areas.

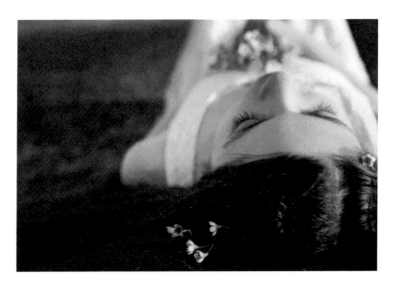

2. Release negative thoughts.

If you start to think any pessimistic thoughts or that you cannot do this, then go back to the previous exercise.

Tell that voice, "Yes, I see that you're just trying to keep me safe. Thank you. But I've got this."

Having done this in the previous exercise, this should be much easier.

3. Connect with your body.

One way to communicate with your body is by placing your hands on the body part that you want to connect to and talking directly to that body part. Let your body know that you are listening. You can tell your body:
>   You can relax now.
>   I am taking care of you.
>   I am open to receive any message that you (or the injured area) would like to share.

4. Ask yourself.

Start with yes/no questions to which you already know the answers and notice how you feel.
>   Is the sky blue?
>   Is the grass red?
>   Do I have a dog?
>   Do I like apples?
>   Is green my favorite color?

You already know the answers, so notice
>   what a "Yes" response feels like;
>   what a "No" response feels like.

Once you start to understand the difference, you can play with questions to which you do not know the answers.

5. Once you start to tap into that wisdom, you can ask more challenging questions.

This skill will improve with time, so be patient with yourself if you do not feel/hear the answers right away.

Sometimes you feel/hear the answer right away; however, sometimes your body will give you the answer later in the day or week, or it will guide you in the direction to find the answers.

You can ask questions like these:
How do I do that?
What do I need to do next?
When will I start?
Why is this good for me?
Where should I go?
Who can help me?
Where can I find the best doctor?
Who is the best person to help me through my healing journey?

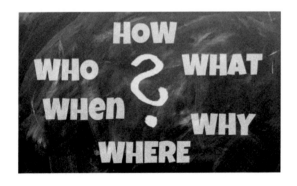

6. Ask with curiosity. Ask with true wonder. Ask with a sense of possibility.

> Be open to seeing with different lenses.
> Be open to trying something new.
> Be open to taking actions.
> Be open to finding yourself.

Notice how you feel.

Well done! You have learned to listen to your inner wisdom, and that will allow you to remember how to self-heal.

> Watch for it.
> Listen for it.
> Ignite it.
> Thank it.
> Act on it.

> The important thing is not to stop questioning. Curiosity has its own reason for existing.
>
> Albert Einstein

6

PLACEBO EFFECT

Your mind is a **powerful healing** tool.

The idea that your brain can convince your body that a treatment is real is called the placebo effect.

The placebo effect is more than positive thinking — believing a treatment or procedure will work. **It is about creating a stronger connection between the brain and body and how they work together** (Harvard Men's Health, 2017).

The placebo effect can cause positive or negative symptoms.

One of the most common theories is that the placebo effect is due to a person's expectations. If a person expects a pill to do something, then it is possible that the body's own chemistry can cause effects similar to what medication might have caused.

I would like to clarify that the fact that the **placebo effect is tied to expectations does not make it imaginary or fake.** Some studies show that there are actual physical changes and pain reduction that occur with the placebo effect (DerSarkissian, 2018).

For example, a study published in the *New England Journal of Medicine,* involving patients with osteoarthritis of the knee, provided strong evidence that arthroscopic surgery was not better than a placebo surgery in improving knee pain and daily function (Moseley, O'Malley, Pete, Menke, Brody, Kuykendall, et al., 2002).

On the flip side, if someone believes that they have a diagnosis, their body can create or amplify many of the symptoms. Again, that does not make the physical changes imaginary or fake. The symptoms are real, the pain is real, the body really feels it, and the body's chemistry actually changes.

As you focus on self-healing, your body relaxes. There is a feeling of hope — just as there is a feeling of hope when someone takes a pill. They believe and trust that the pill will help and that it will make a difference.

The pharmaceutical companies definitely do not want you to believe that **your body is wired to self-heal**.

We have a perfect system that identifies, filters, and destroys anything that does not serve us, and eliminates it from our body. It self-regulates to accommodate our age, our weight, our lifestyle. All the hormones are designed to dance around each other and balance each other. All joints, ligaments and muscles work in perfect synchronicity to facilitate graceful movement.

The placebo effect is just part of the body's healing technique.

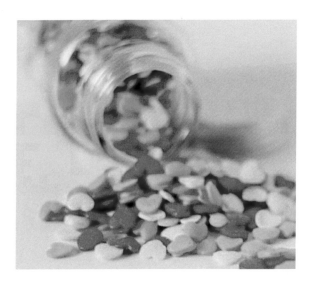

Even when something is not perfect, the body learns to adapt and thrive.

Do you not believe me?

Consider the athletes with impairments that participate in the Paralympic Games.

All you need to do is learn how to tap into that power and allow the body to do what the body knows — heal!

Ana Marinho

HOW CAN I ACTIVATE
THE PLACEBO EFFECT
TO HEAL?

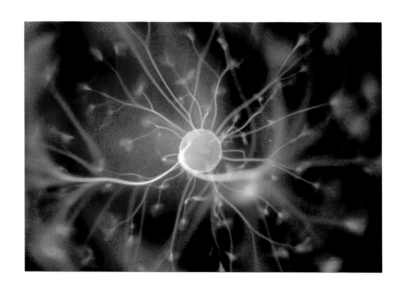

Exercise: Ignite Your Inner Healer

Every day, for one week, sit comfortably in a quiet place.
Notice how you are feeling.
Notice how your body feels.
Repeat the previous steps as needed.

1. Take a few deep breaths and notice your body.

Bring attention to the areas of your health that you would like to improve. Notice your discomfort, pain, tightness, temperature, emotions...

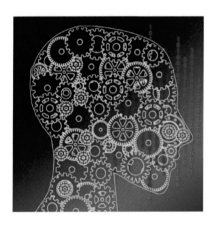

2. Imagine a perfect body.

Imagine your body working in synchronicity — every organ, every cell, every bone, all working together.

It is just like the gears of a clock. Everything is working perfectly.

Each organ is doing its job. Each muscle is strong and healthy. Every joint has enough lubrication and is gliding smoothly.

Imagine your body healthy and happy.
What would it look like to live pain- free?
What would it feel like to have no limitation?
What would it feel like to have a healthy body?

3. Take your 'magic pill'.

Imagine yourself taking a 'magic pill' that will resolve your specific problem. You can even use empty capsules if you want. Maybe ask your body what you can add to the capsule (like honey, essential oils, etc.).

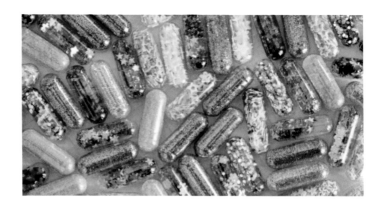

4. Feel the 'magic pill' working.

Visualize that 'magic pill' entering your body and working exactly where you need. It is the best medication, and one that does not have any side effects. Enjoy the feeling.

5. Be gentle with yourself.

Allow the body to remember how to heal. It may take a few seconds or it may take a few days. The speed at which it occurs is perfect for *you.* Your response is perfect for *you.* Be curious. Trust. Surrender.

Be open to seeing with different lenses.
Be open to trying something new.
Be open to taking actions.
Be open to finding yourself.

Notice how you feel before and after.
Notice what changes in the coming days.

Well done, dear one! You have just allowed your inner healer to remember how to self-heal.

Watch for it.
Listen for it.
Ignite it.
Thank it.
Act on it.

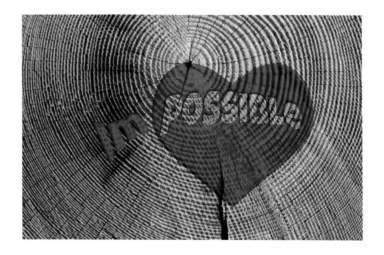

The greatest wealth is health.

Virgil

SUMMARY

How to ignite your inner healer:

Start to change your thoughts, allowing the brain to rewire itself, creating new neuropathways (neuroplasticity).

Start to notice new possibilities around you.

Listen to your body wisdom. Ask your body what it needs to create the best environment to heal.

Focus on the results that you expect (placebo effect).

Trust and allow the body to heal.

Remember *you* have the power.

Be curious, laugh, have fun, trust, dance, sing, experiment, allow, play...

LOTUS FLOWER'S SYMBOLISM

The lotus flower is an aquatic plant, viewed as a sacred and powerful symbol by many ancient cultures. The lotus flower offers countless meanings and interpretations.

Anybody who has ever seen a lotus emerging from a dirty pond cannot help but see the beauty that this exquisite plant provides.

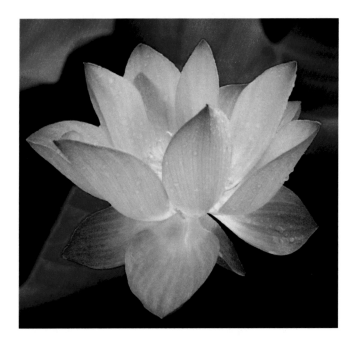

The lotus flower grows from the bottom of streams and muddy ponds to rise above the water and bloom. The lotus flower is proof that a bold, bright life can arise from the darkest of places.

A Buddhist proverb says that the lotus flower blooms most beautifully from the deepest and thickest mud. This is such a great metaphor for life as well. Just like the lotus, we too have the ability to rise from the mud.

Every difficult situation that is hard to navigate can ultimately lead to beautiful outcomes and help us to grow into even better human beings.

So, next time that you face a challenge, remember there is always a choice.

You can choose to take no action and remain stagnant in the mud...

Or you can be like a lotus flower.

You can make the best of your situation and rise above the mud.

Be Like the Lotus Flower!

SHARE THE LOVE

If you enjoyed the teachings in this book and found them valuable, I would very much appreciate your paying it forward to your like-minded friends and family members.

It is easy to give this book as a gift or write a positive review on Amazon.

Let me know if there is any other way I can help you. Simply email me at ana@behealthywithana.com.

I hope to be hearing from you soon!

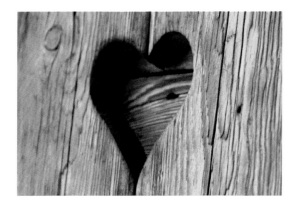

REFERENCES

Belluck, P. (2013). "Common Knee Surgery Does Very Little for Some, Study Suggests". Retrieved from https://www.nytimes.com/2013/12/26/health/common-knee-surgery-does-very-little-for-some-study-suggests.html

CBHS. (2017). "This is why optimism is better than positive thinking". Retrieved from CBHS Health Fund: https://www.cbhs.com.au/health-well-being-blog/blog-article/2017/10/02/this-is-why-optimism-is-better-than-positive-thinking

Cremaldi, J., & Bhushan, B. (2018). "Bioinspired self-healing materials: lessons from nature". Retrieved from *Beilstein Journal of Nanotechnology*: https://www.ncbi.nlm.nih.gov/pmc/articles/PMC5870156/

DerSarkissian, C. (2018). "What Is the Placebo Effect?" . Retrieved from WebMD: https://www.webmd.com/pain-management/what-is-the-placebo-effect#1

Harvard Men's Health Watch (2017). "The power of the placebo effect". Retrieved from *Harvard Men's Health Watch*: https://www.health.harvard.edu/mental-health/the-power-of-the-placebo-effect

Hecht, D. (2013). "The Neural Basis of Optimism and Pessimism". Retrieved from *Experimental Neurobiology*: https://www.ncbi.nlm.nih.gov/pmc/articles/PMC3807005/

Milner, C. (2018). "Your Self-Healing Body". Retrieved from *The Epoch Times*: https://www.theepochtimes.com/your-self-healing-body-2_2561958.html

Moseley, B., O'Malley, K., Pete, N., Menke, T., Brody, B., Kuykendall, D., . . . Wray, N. (2002). "A Controlled Trial of Arthroscopic Surgery for Osteoarthritis of the Knee". Retrieved from *The New England Journal of Medicine*: https://www.nejm.org/doi/full/10.1056/NEJMoa013259

Schroeder, M. (2016). "Death by Prescription". Retrieved from *U.S. News*: https://health.usnews.com/health-news/patient-advice/articles/2016-09-27/the-danger-in-taking-prescribed-medications

Swart, T. (2018). "The 4 Underlying Principles of Changing Your Brain". Retrieved from *Forbes*: https://www.forbes.com/sites/taraswart/2018/03/27/the-4-underlying-principles-to-changing-your-brain/#4bc7d6535a71

U.S. Centers for Medicare & Medicaid Services. (2016). "National Health Expenditures 2016 Highlights". Retrieved from U.S. Centers for Medicare & Medicaid Services: https://www.cms.gov/Research-Statistics-Data-and-Systems/Statistics-Trends-and-Reports/NationalHealthExpendData/downloads/highlights.pdf

UCSB. (2013). "How many cells do we have in our body?". Retrieved from https://scienceline.ucsb.edu/getkey.php?key=3926

Williams, Y. (2018). "Optimistic vs Pessimistic Thinking". Retrieved from https://study.com/academy/lesson/optimistic-vs-pessimistic-thinking.html

Some images used in this book are from the author's private gallery. Other images are from www.unsplash.com and www.pixabay.com and are made available under the Free Creative Commons License.

The information provided in this book is not intended to diagnose, treat, cure or prevent any disease. This book is not intended as a substitute for appropriate medical care.
It is intended as a sharing of knowledge and information from the author's research and experience.

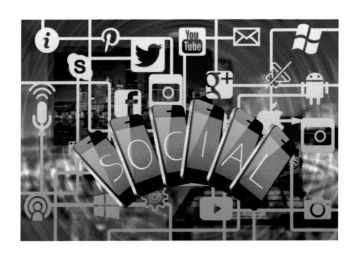

You can use the hashtag **#IgniteYourInnerHealer**
on Social Media

Facebook:
www.facebook.com/BeHealthyWithAna/

Instagram:
www.instagram.com/be_healthy_ana_marinho/

YouTube: Be Healthy - Ana Marinho

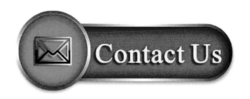

Be Healthy, LLC

Ana Marinho

Web: www.behealthywithana.com

Phone: 424-225-2313

Email: ana@behealthywithana.com

ABOUT THE AUTHOR

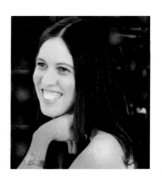

Over her ten-year career, Ana Marinho has helped hundreds of patients to ignite the power of their own self-healing.

As a physical therapist, intuitive healer and health coach, Ana has a unique background and experience across a wide range of self-healing disciplines, allowing her to tap into both the scientific and the alternative aspects of healing simultaneously.

In fact, when Ana was diagnosed with a chronic disease, she restored her own health using the same techniques outlined in this book — with no doctors and with no drugs.

BONUS
Want some extra support?

This book is just the beginning of an amazing journey. If you want to go deeper, working hand in hand with Ana is the fast track for accessing your inner healing.

Clients have raved about the remarkable benefits of her one-on-one sessions. If you want this extra level of support, schedule your first appointment now and get a 30 percent discount.

Schedule your appointment today!

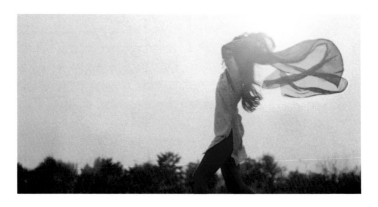

Sessions with Ana are offered online by video conference or in person at Ana's office in Charlotte, North Carolina.

30% OFF
your first appointment
Discount code: #Ignite

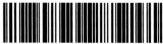
50539306R00042

Made in the USA
Columbia, SC
08 February 2019